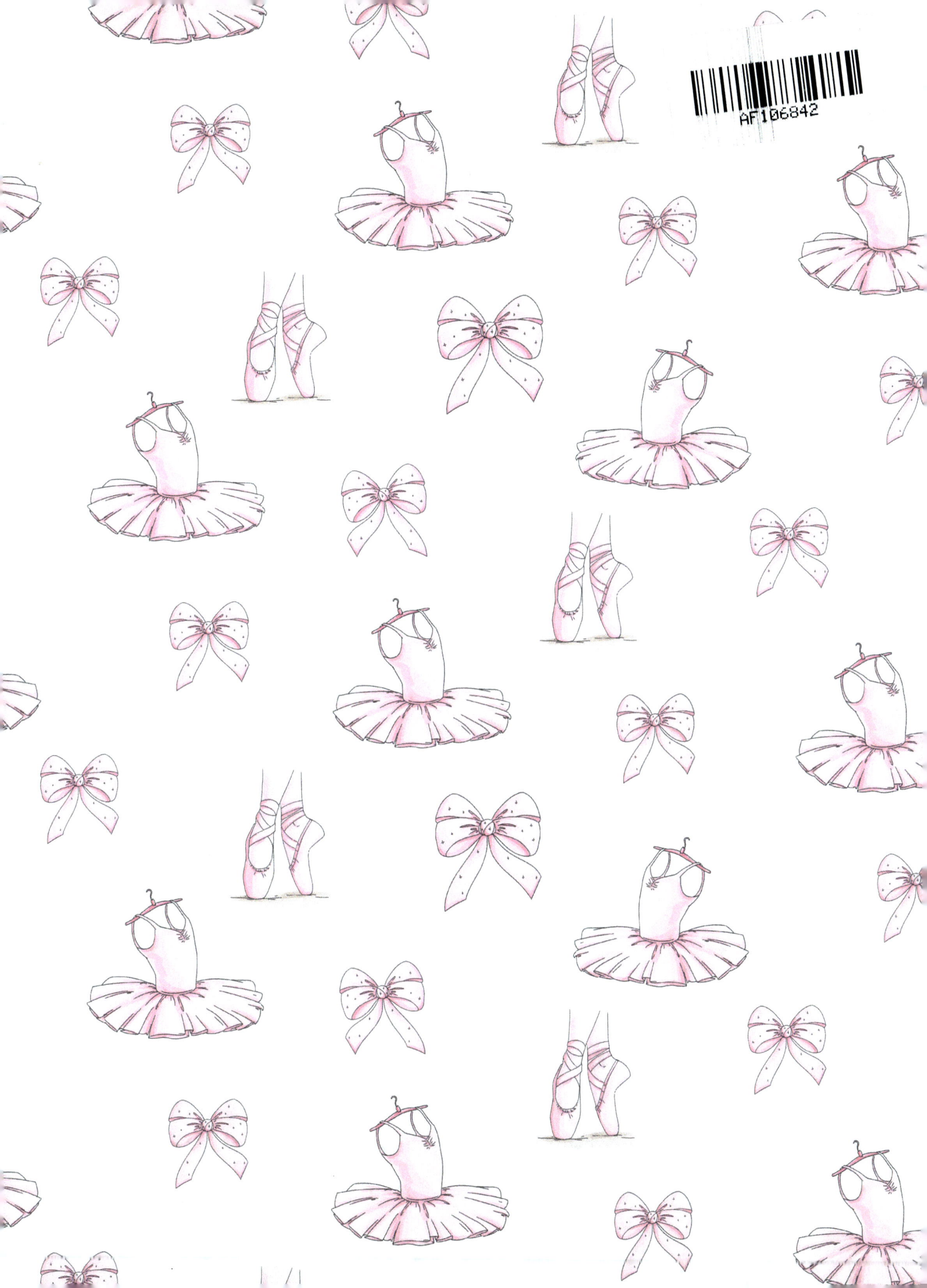

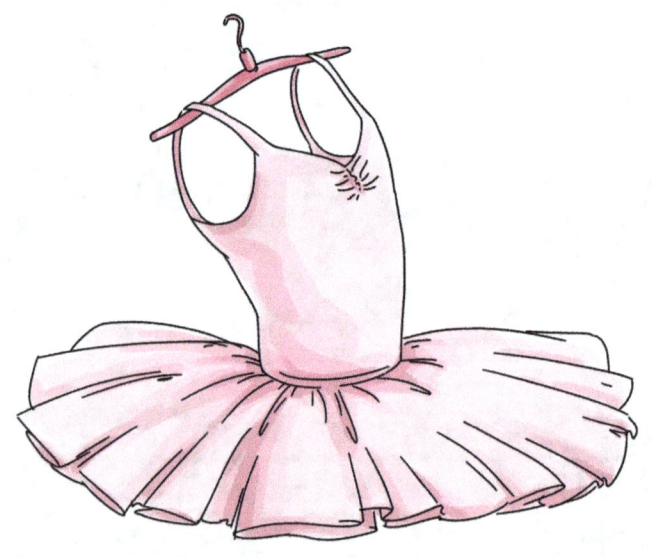

Copyright© 2022 by Anne-Marie Pos-Terlouw

All rights reserved. No part of this book may be reproduced or used in any manner without written permission of copyright owner except for the use of quotations in a book review.

Learn Ballet
with **Miss Zoey**

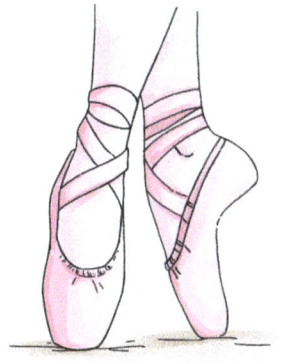

Anne-Marie Pos-Terlouw

Illustrations by
Erzsebet Zsofia Ferencz

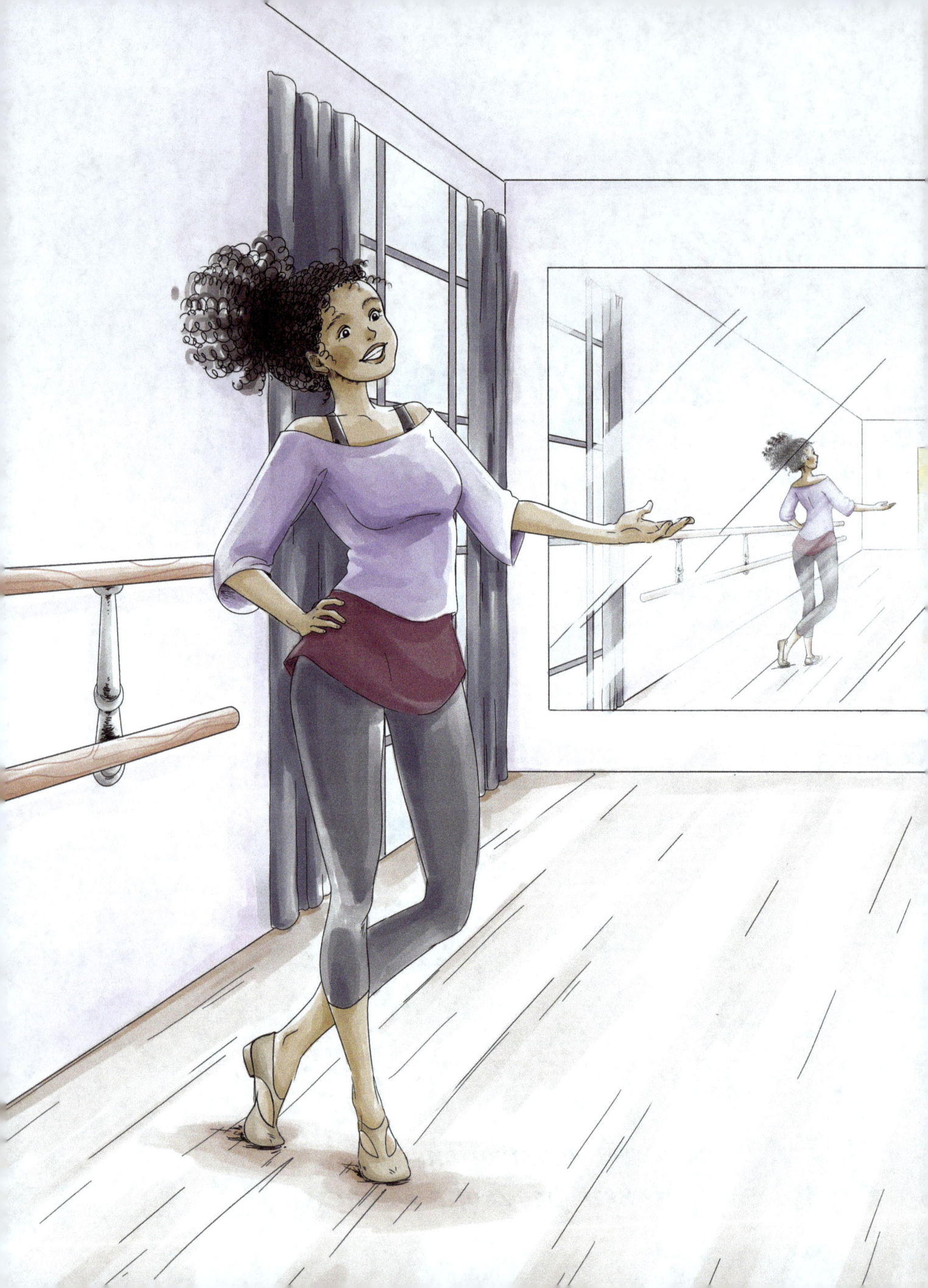

Hi,
I am Miss Zoey, and I am going to teach you the basics of ballet.

Anyone can do ballet. Did you know that? It doesn't matter if you are a girl or a boy, what you look like, or how old you are. If you like to dance ballet, then you just do it.

A few people become professional ballet dancers. Many more people dance ballet every week, as a hobby. Just because they like it, and it is fun. And that is what it is all about, fun in ballet dancing.

Different countries around the world have several ballet methods. But in general, a lot is the same. There are small differences in names of the postures and steps, but all the names are in French. It depends on your ballet teacher how you are taught. So, keep in mind that a ballet class from another teacher is not immediately wrong, but slightly different. And that's fine.

Let's go through the basics together!

Chapter 1: What do you need?

You can start in leggings, a shirt and bare feet or socks. Later you can get things like a leotard, tights, ballet leggings, a ballet skirt, leg warmers, and flat ballet shoes. After years of training, you can talk to your teacher about buying and starting to dance on pointe shoes. This is something for advanced ballet dancers.

In the dance school we practice at the ballet barre. This is a stick we put our hands on to help us with our balance. At home you can use the back of a chair, the back of your sofa or stand next to the counter in your kitchen. Even putting your hand against a wall is fine. Make sure you have some free space around you to move. Be careful not to hit a piece of furniture with an arm or leg.

It takes some effort and creativity, but if you really want to practice and dance at home, you can. Ask your teacher for some tips. At the dance school we also give online ballet classes. And we see that practicing at home can go very well
if you really want to.

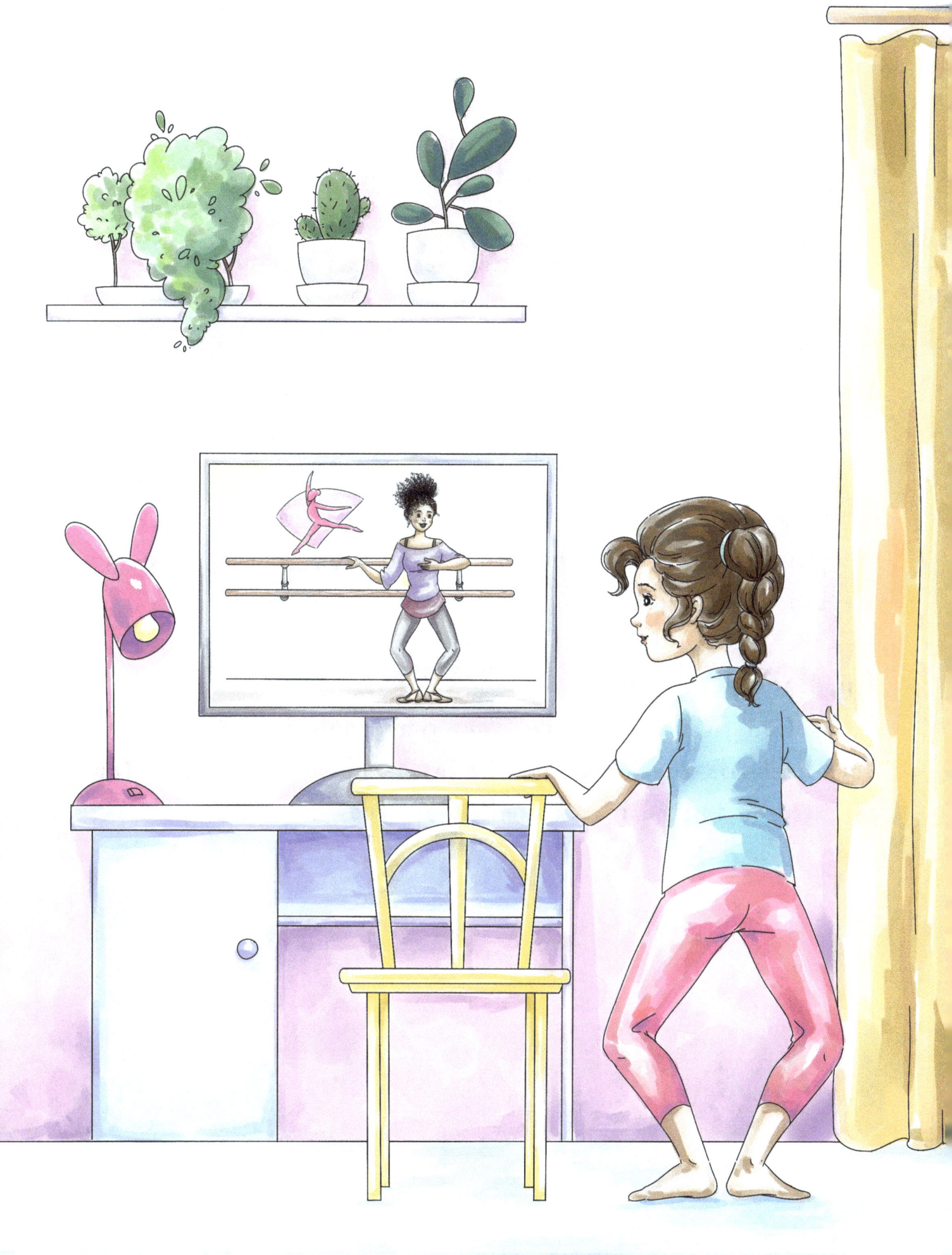

Chapter 2: The Six-Foot Positions.

There are six-foot positions. Here are the first three.

First position:
Turn your legs out in the hips. Put your heels together. Your knees and feet are pointing outward.

Second position:
Put your feet one and a half foot apart. Now you are standing in the second position. Keep your balance in the middle.

Third position:
Go back to first position. Put your right foot in front of the left. Your heel fits snugly against the inside of your left foot. You can also do this position with the left foot in front.

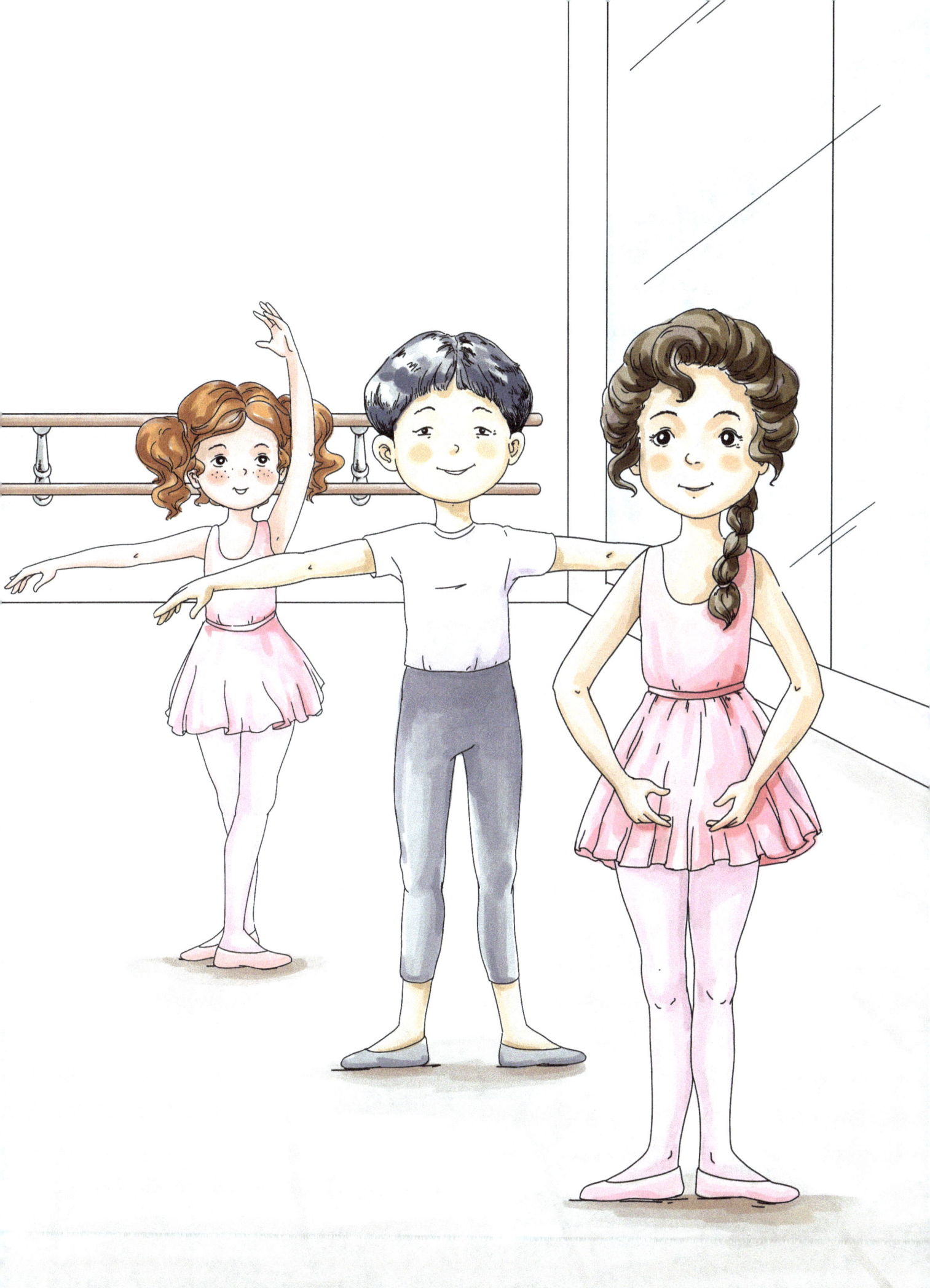

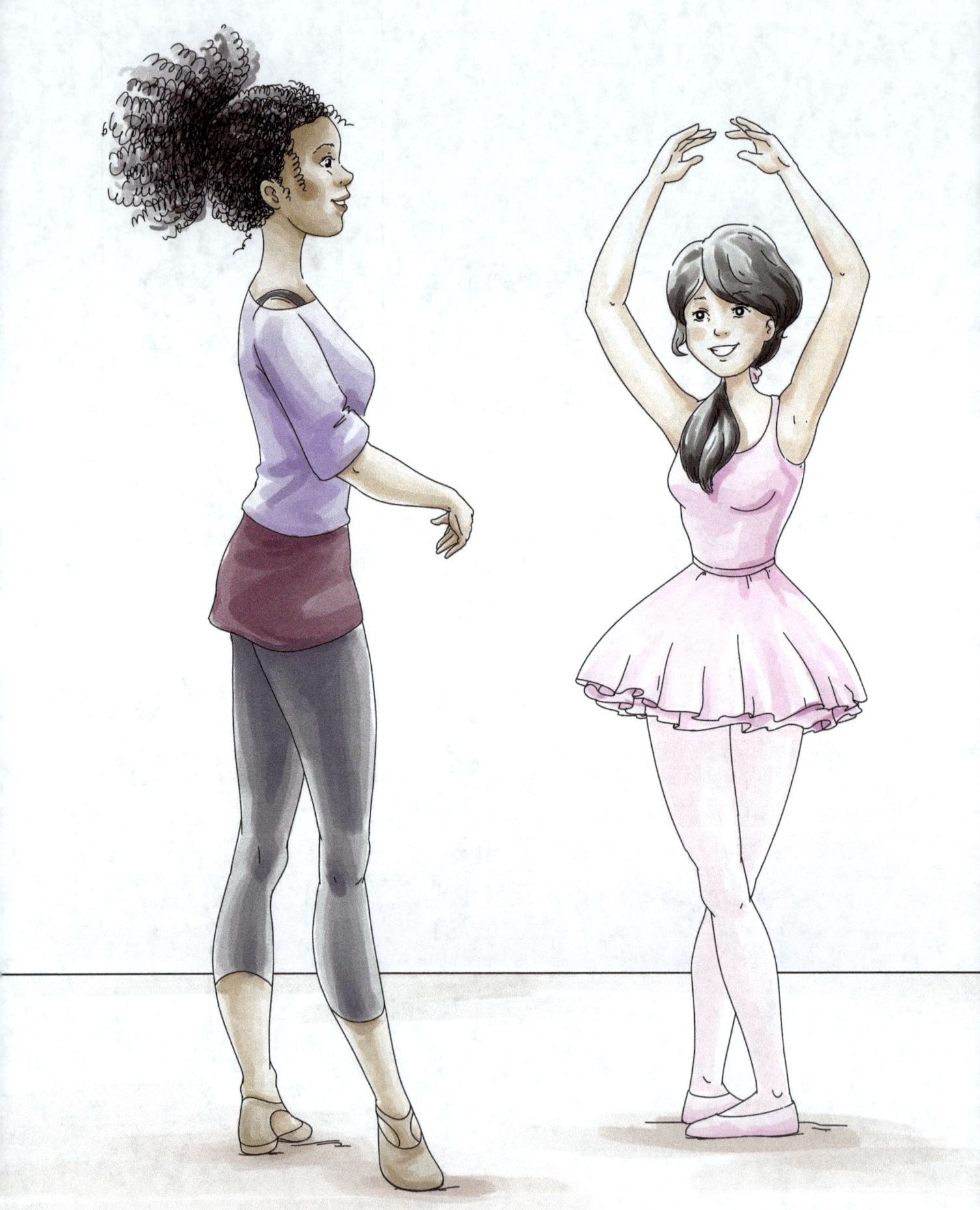

Fourth position:
Back to the first position. Go straight forward with your right foot and put it on the floor. You want to have a foot and a half between your front and your back foot. Stand exactly in the middle. Keep your hip bones in one line and straight forward.

Fifth position:
Back to the third position. To stand in the fifth position, now cross your front foot and leg slightly over. Your heel is now next to the big toe of your back foot. You are now super crossed with your legs. Yes, this is the most difficult position.

Sixth position: You stand with your feet next to each other, your toes and knees pointing forward.

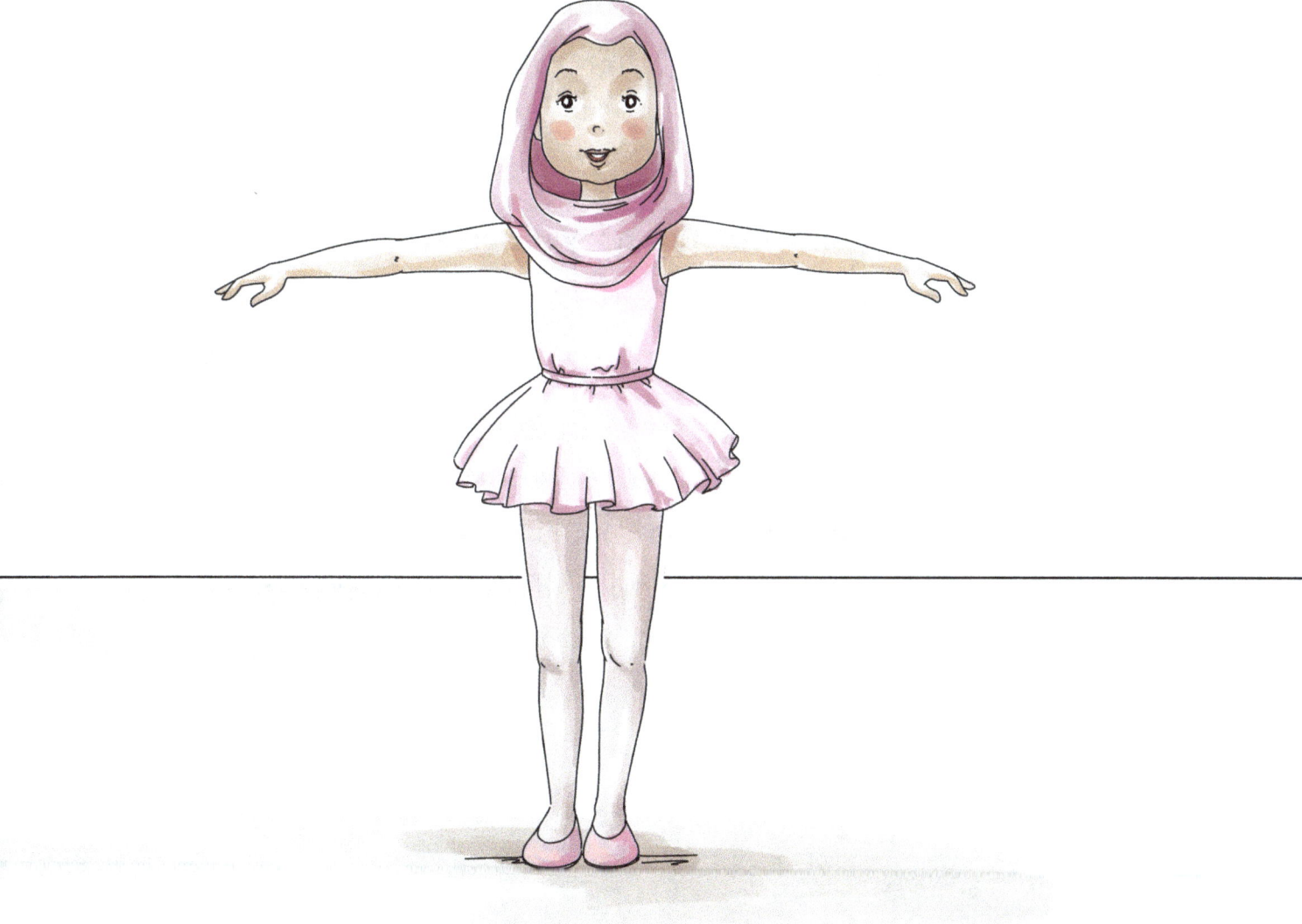

Chapter 3: How does a ballet dancer stand?

Before we start dancing, you must stand for a moment.
Yes, I know, you want to start dancing right away. But go ahead anyway because it is important to understand and feel which muscles to use.

Stand in the sixth foot position. Pretend to close the zipper of a pair of jeans that are a little bit too tight. Do you feel that? Your belly button goes back, and your pelvis goes down. Your stomach muscles are going up. You are already standing taller. And your muscles are activated. Do you also feel your buttock muscles working now?
Make sure you don't squeeze too much, because then you can hardly move anymore.

Now pretend a string from the top of your head runs along your neck, further down along your spine and all the way to your tailbone.
At your head the string goes up to the ceiling. At your tailbone the string goes down into the floor. Have you ever seen a marionette? Just think about that. Check if your shoulders are on top of the hips. Think of a blocktower and you want to put every piece right on top of the next. Nice! Now we know how a ballet dancer can stand so beautifully tall.

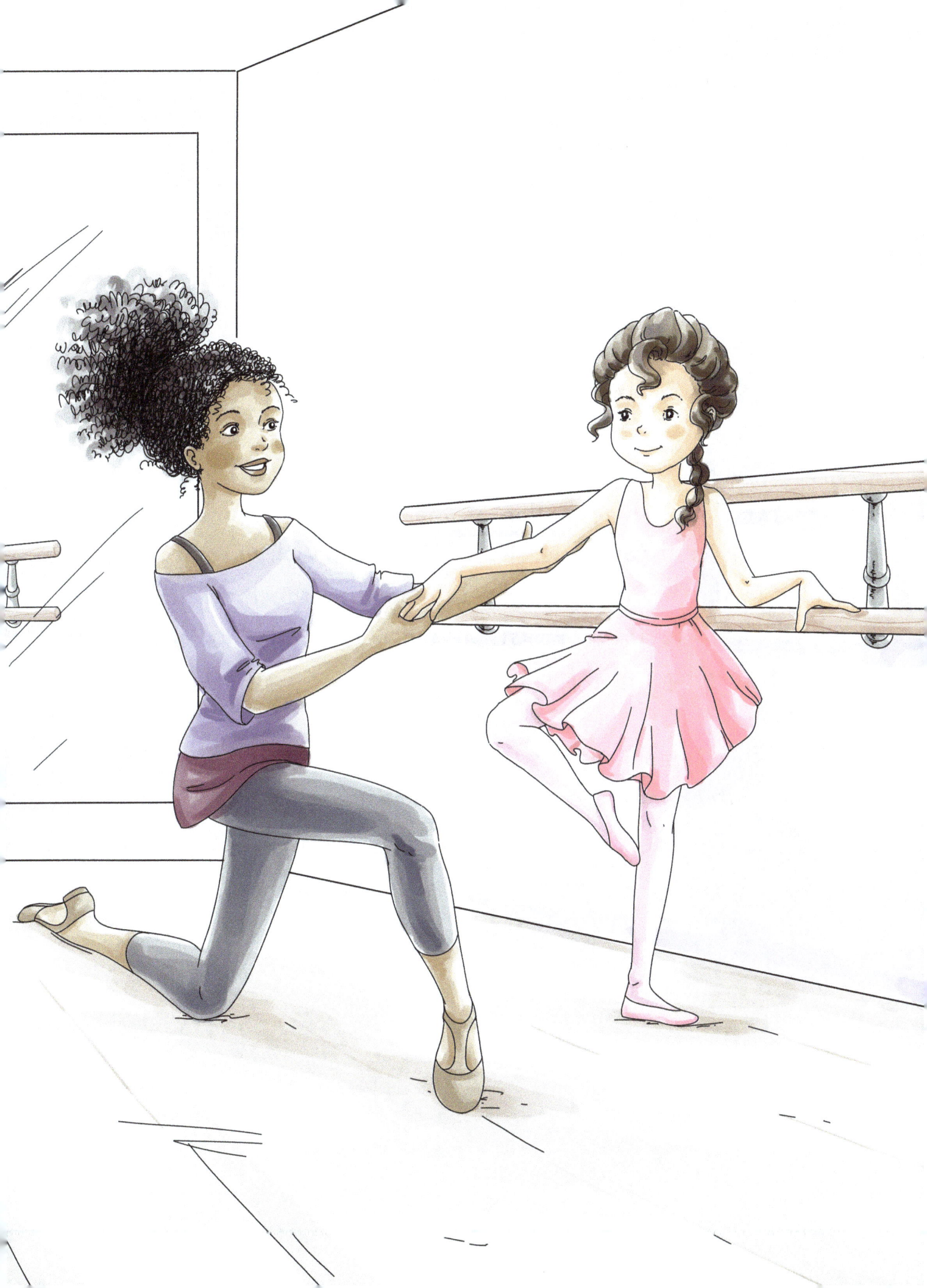

Chapter 4: Turnout and flexibility.

For the foot positions you need to open and rotate your legs. In ballet we call that turnout. Why do we turn our legs out in ballet? Well, then we have even more freedom of movement than when the legs are parallel or even turned in. And when you start to lift or throw your legs up, they can go higher.

Stand on your left leg and turn out (open and close) your right leg. Do you feel the turning motion of the leg in your hip socket? If it is a little difficult to do, go ahead and try it with your arms in your shoulder joint. This is easier. By turning the arm, the palm of the hand will move to an open position and close again. We can do the same with our legs in the hip sockets.

You hold this turned-out position by activating your lower abdomen muscles, buttock muscles and inner thigh muscles.

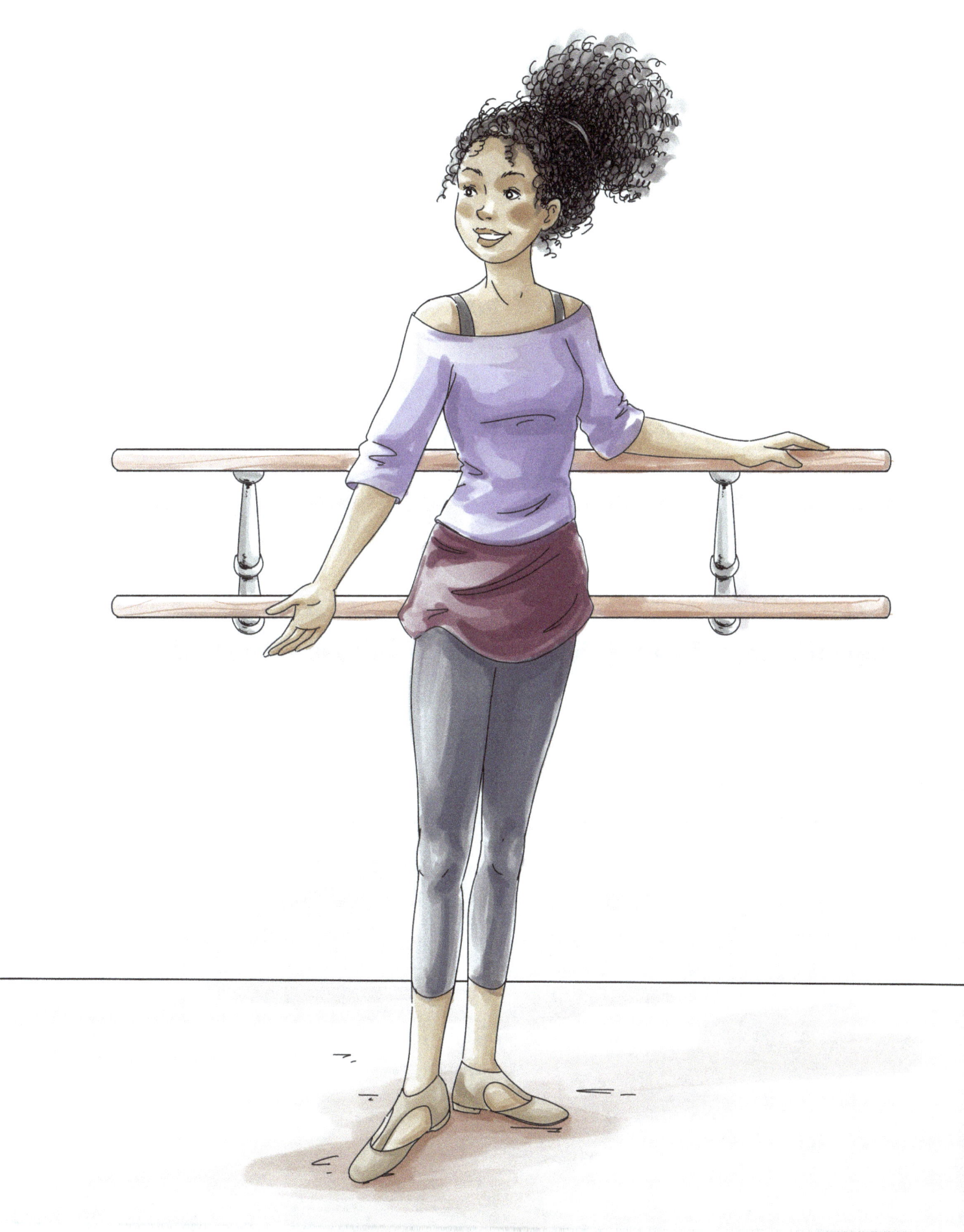

You can practice flexibility by sitting on the floor, putting your legs out in front of you and now opening both up. This position is also called the second position although you are sitting on the floor. Your legs are turned out, so your knees will point up to the ceiling. Try to stretch your legs all the way out to your toes.

In this position you can practice achieving a sideways split. Practice gently, don't hurt yourself. Sit in the position and feel your muscles in the legs stretch gently. When you become more comfortable, you can go ahead and open the legs a little more. Every time a little more, until you have your sideways split.

To practice your forward split you also need your turnout. The more turned out, the easier it is for you to go sit down in the split with one leg forward and one leg back.

Great! Now let's continue with the arm positions.

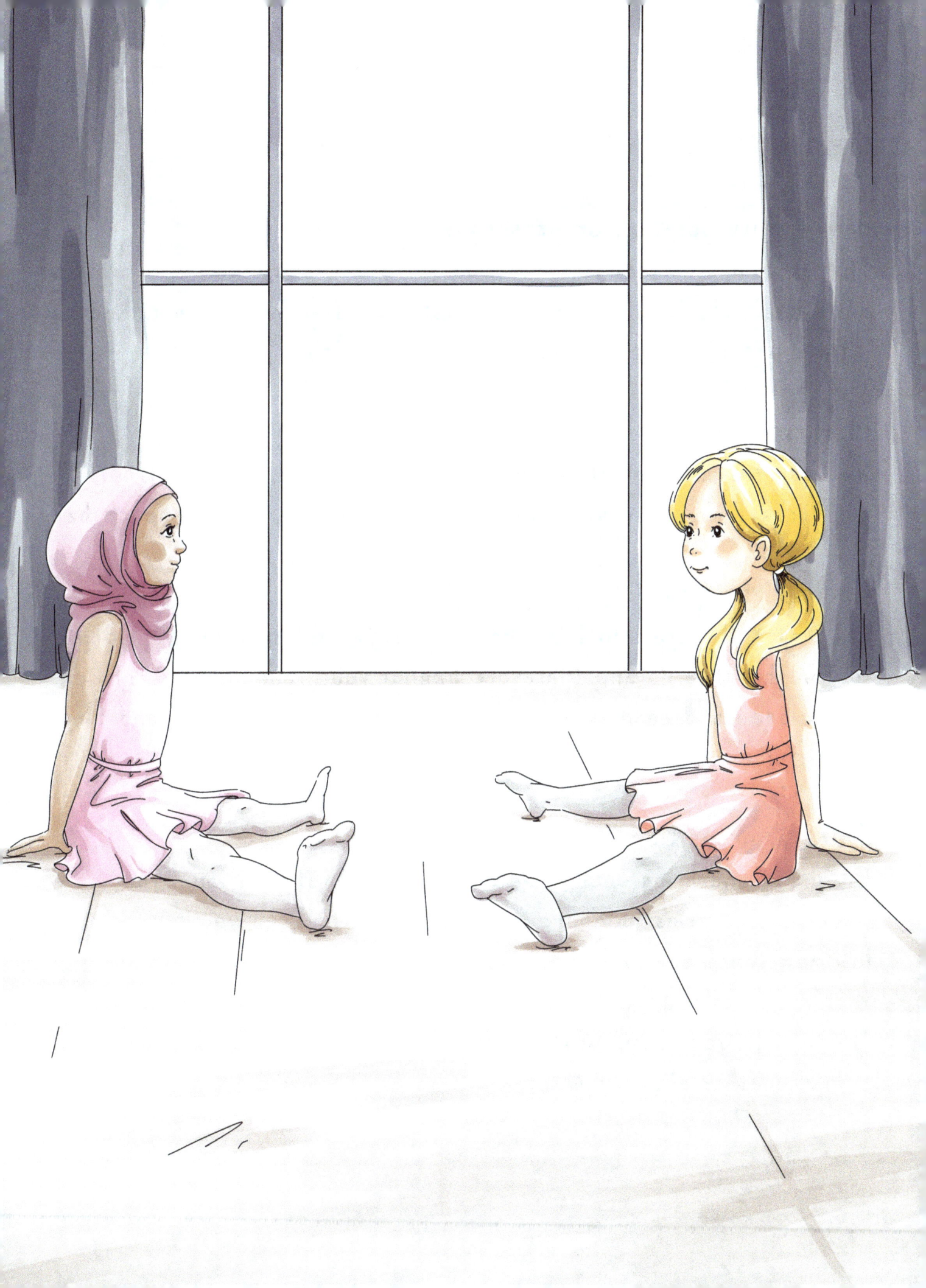

Chapter 5: The 3 Arm Position of the Vaganova Method.

Preparatory position or bras bas:
This is your start and end position for every exercise. Your arms are down, and rounded. The elbows, wrists and fingers are soft. Keep a little space between your hands and your thighs.

First arm position:
We keep the arms nicely rounded and raise them, right in front of your breast bone and your ribs. Like holding a very large beach ball.

Second arm position:
Let's open the arms to the side. Be careful not to bring your arms too much outwards and therefore behind you. Your shoulder blades are relaxed and open. Keep your shoulders, elbows, wrists and fingers beautifully aligned. Don't let the elbows drop.

Third arm position:
Go ahead and bring your arms back to the first position. From here we bring the arms up above your head. Try to keep your shoulders low and your neck long. You want to hinge your arms up, think of that marionette we talked about earlier. Make a beautiful picture frame with your arms around your head. The hands and fingers come together above your crown.

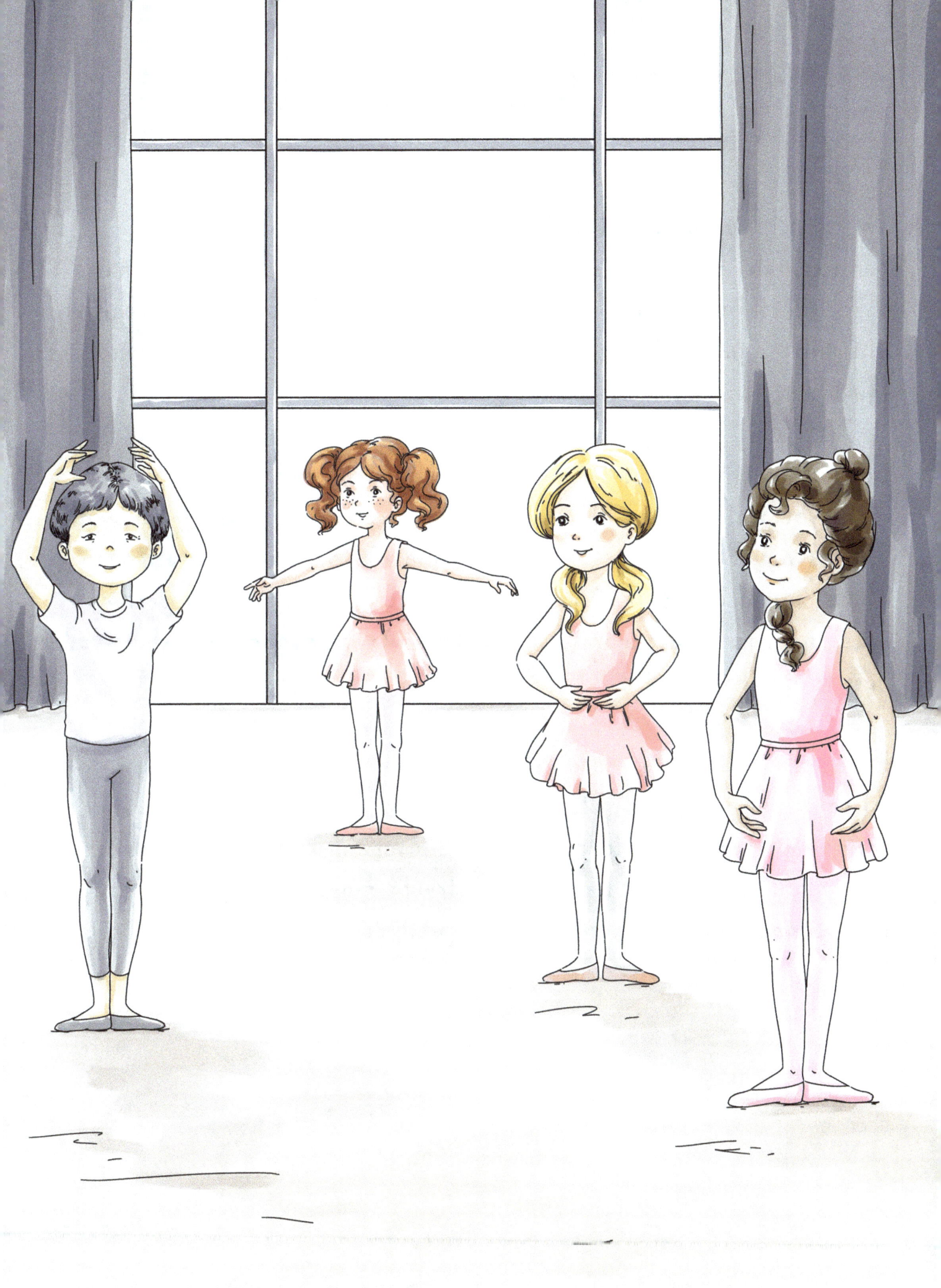

There are two more extra positions in other ballet methods. For example, in RAD, Cecchetti or Bournonville methods. In that case, the third position above your head is called the fifth position. The third and fourth positions are combinations of first, second and third arm positions.

Don't worry if you can't remember it all right away. In the ballet class you will practice the positions separately, but also in movement. This is called a port de bras. Which means to carry your arms. There are also different port de bras such as preparatory port de bras and first and second port de bras. Your teacher will show you how to do those.

Here is a tip: Try to recreate the arm positions while looking into a mirror. Long neck and relaxed muscles in the neck. You can still move your head. Shoulders are low and open. Your shoulderblades are not pulled together, but open. Now try to move from position to position, connecting the photos. Lovely, well done!

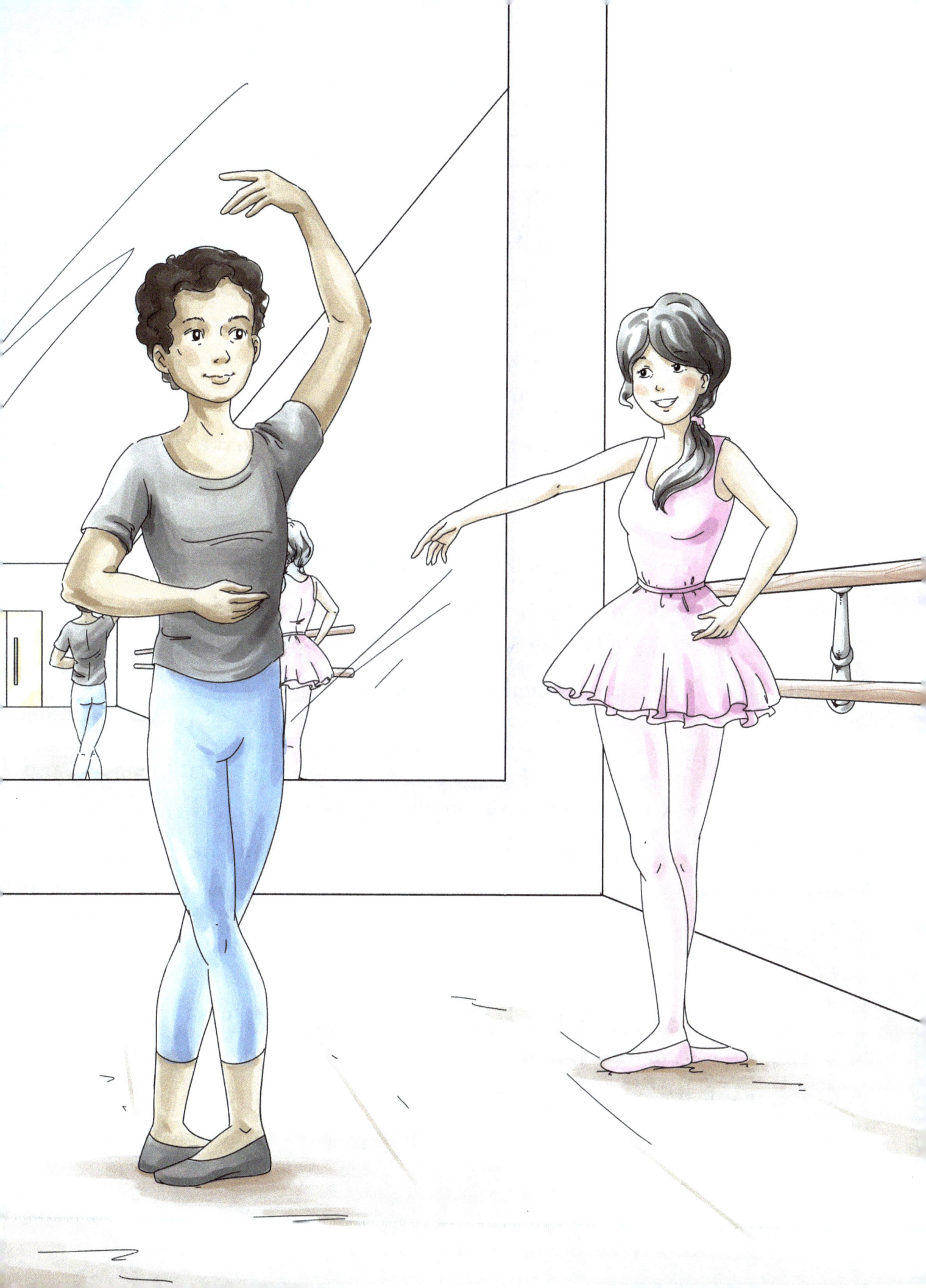

Chapter 6: Hands, fingers, head and shoulders in ballet.

The movement of the head and shoulders with your ballet steps is called 'épaulement'. This helps to make the movements softer or more dynamic, depending on the steps and the character of your dance. Using épaulement makes it complete and alive.

Try to apply a freely moving head, neck, and shoulders as soon as possible, as it is very difficult to learn and apply later. Your teacher will help you out with the correct movements and make sure you are not overdoing it.

Your core (abdomen or stomach muscles) is strong and in place. From that strong center of the body, the arms, shoulders, neck, and head can move freely. Relax your neck muscles and shoulders. The muscles in the face should also relax.

The fingers should always be in alignment with your wrist, elbow, and shoulder. The positions are very much rounded. Even when we make an allongé movement, a movement where we extend the fingers and hands to move to another position, the wrist and elbow joints are soft and not overstretched.

In the rounded positions the fingers are somewhat together. They are long and soft. And the thumb is soft and a little in, towards the midsection of the second finger. You don't have to put the thumb directly on the finger, leave a little bit of space between the thumb and second finger.

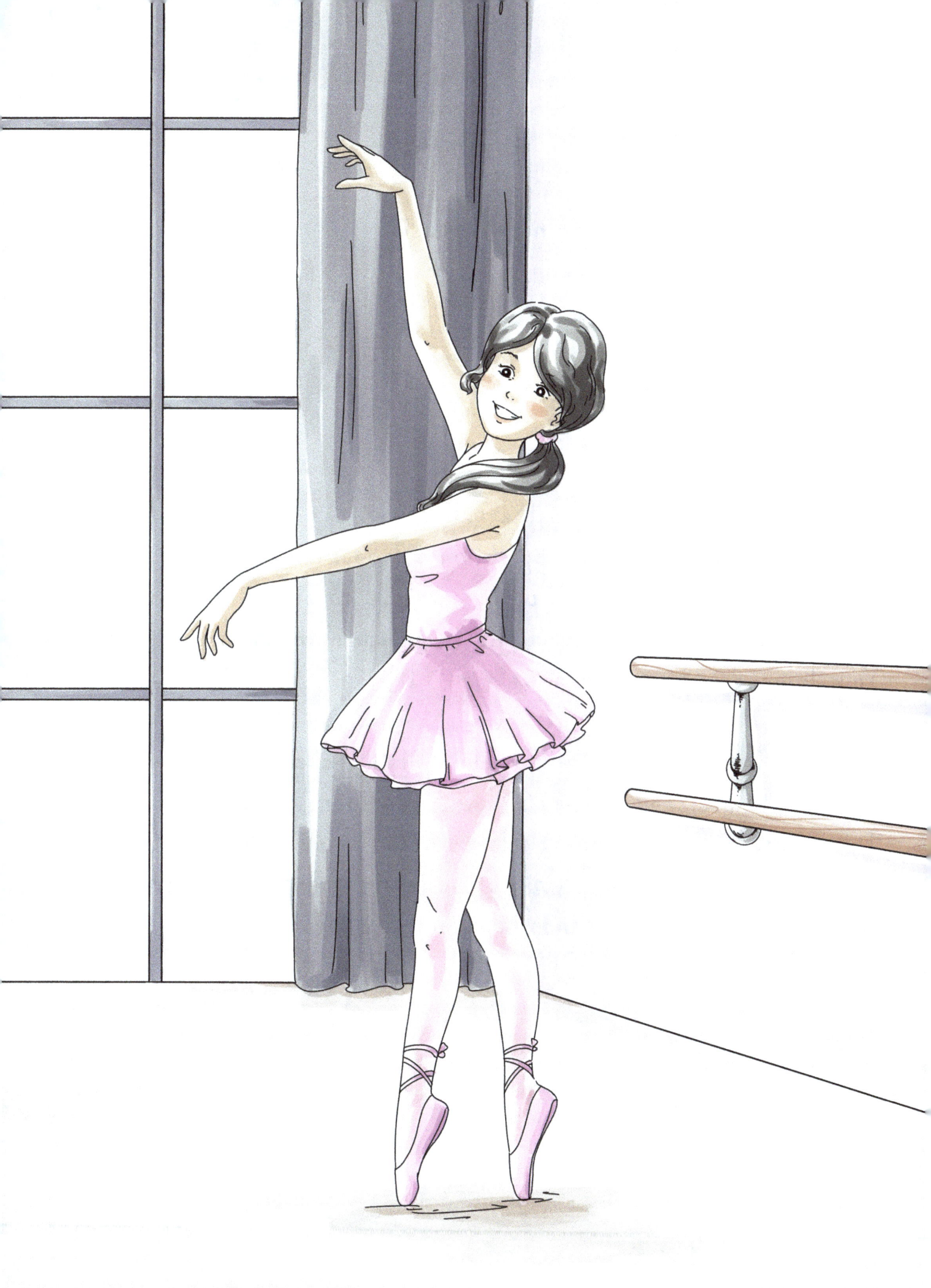

Introduction to the 3 basic movements

All ballet steps consist of these 3 basic, but very important, movements.

1. Plié
2. Elevé or/and relevé
3. Tendu

For example, you cannot do the ballet step pas de bourrée without plié, relevé and tendu. A preparation for a pirouette always has a tendu, a plié and then goes up to a relevé to start the turn.
A ballet jump starts out of a plié to go up in the air via a relevé. Your landing is back in a plié.

On the following pages I will explain what these three basic movements are. You will learn how to do them correctly.
These three are the building blocks of so many steps and ballet combinations. It will help you get better in ballet and have more fun because you understand these building blocks.

Let's start!

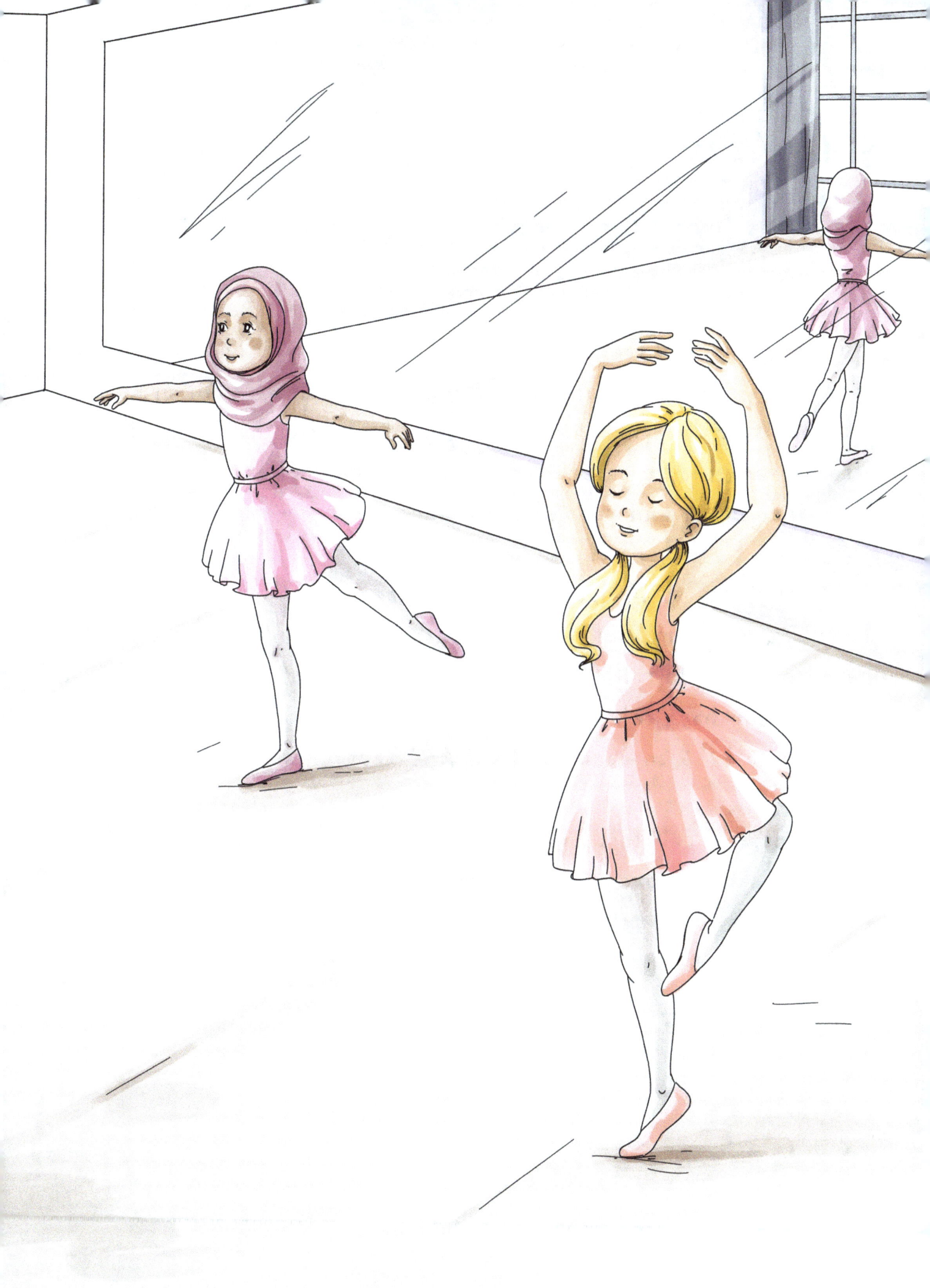

Chapter 7: Plié

Plié means folded. It is a movement where you fold or bend in the knee joints.

The demi plié is exactly the same in all foot positions. You bend in your knees and ankles and go straight down and straight up. Keep your heels on the floor and press your feet into the floor when you stretch back up. Be careful not to move your pelvis back or forwards. Keep the pelvis, and your hips, in place.

Think of a beautiful, open diamond shape when you plié. Because you are using your turn out, the knees are pointing over your toes.
Be careful not to roll forward over the inside of your feet. This will indicate you have let go of your muscles. Use your inner thigh muscles to keep an open position. And keep all toes on the floor.

Well done. We call this knee bend a demi pié, a halve bend.
There is also a movement that we call the big bend, the grand plié.
Let's see on the next page.

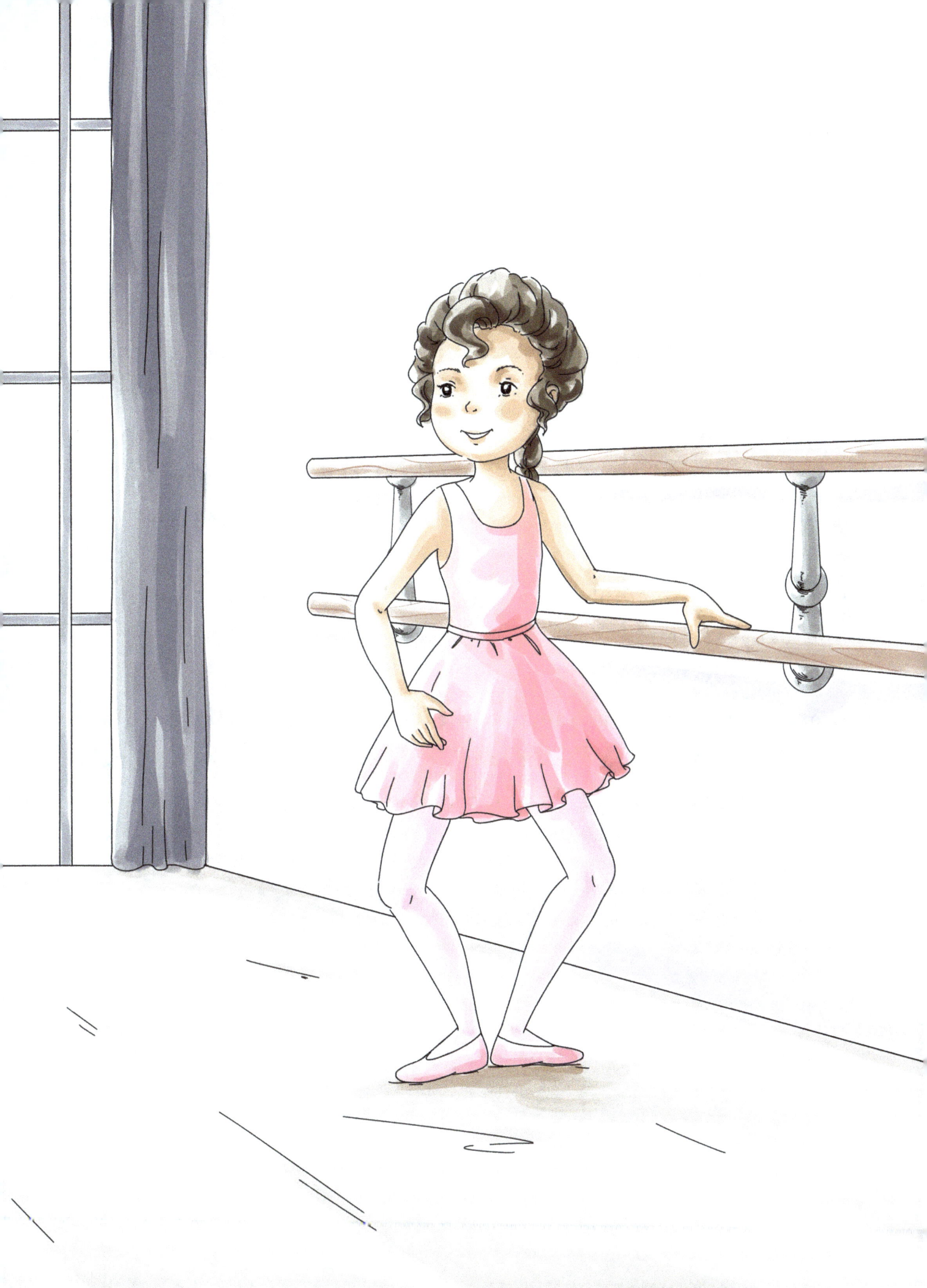

How to do a grand plié.

Stand up straight in the third position. Start with a demi plié.
Go to the point where you can keep your heels on the floor.
Now gently let the heels come loose. Pay attention not to lift your
heels, just let them come loose while bending even further down.
Stay upright with your body. Your shoulders stay above your hips.
Your pelvis stays straight and your tailbone down to the floor.
When you arrive at your deepest point, start to move back up to the
demi plié. And from there you stretch all the way up again.

Try to move as smoothly as possible and be careful not to sit
at the deepest point.

The grand plié goes the same in the first, third, fourth, fifth and
sixth foot positions. In the second foot position the heels remain
firmly in the ground and do not come loose.

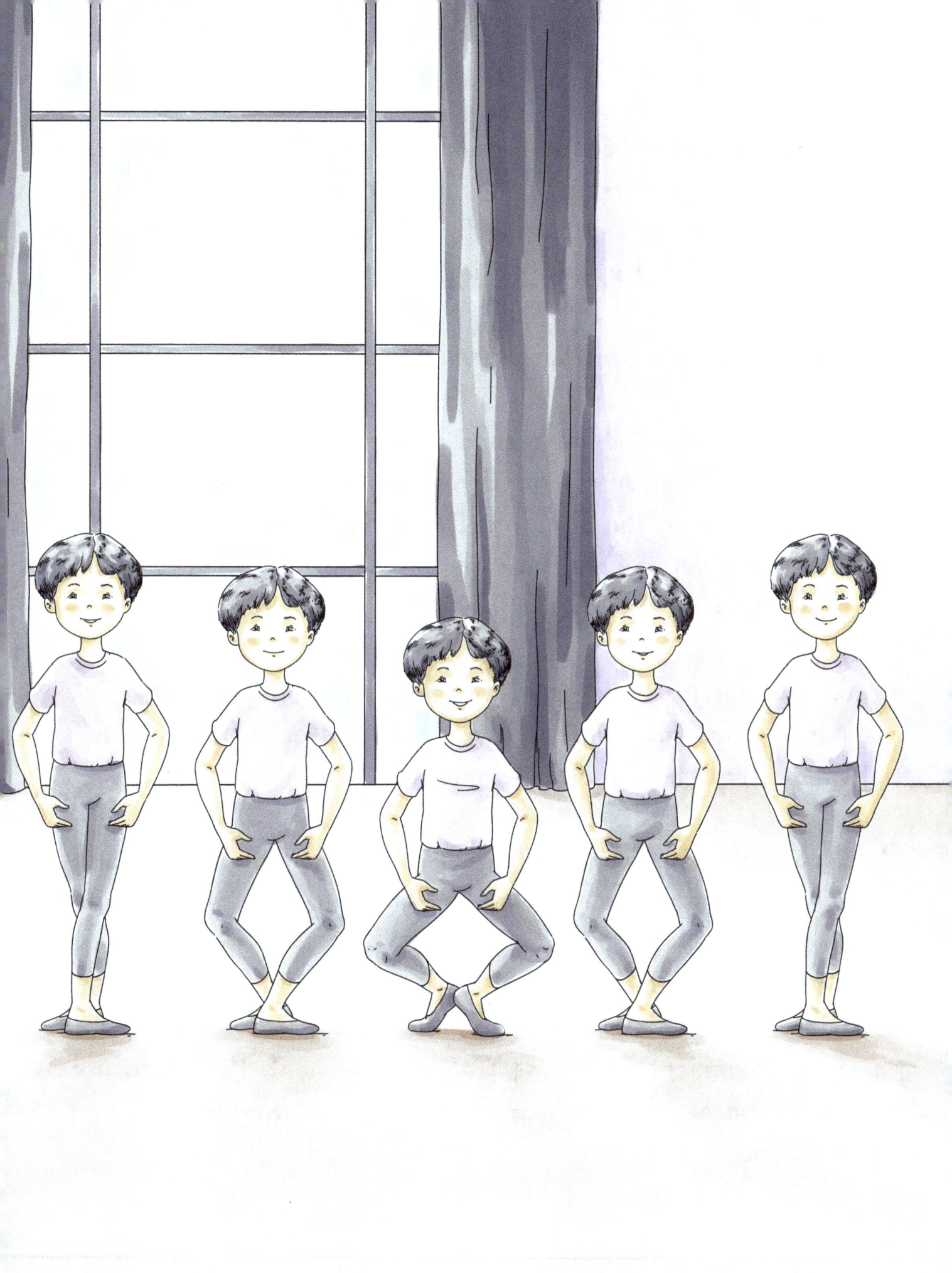

While doing a demi plié, the arms can go in different positions. For example, if you are going to turn pirouettes later in class, you will practice opening and closing the arms in the first and second arm position at the barre with pliés.

Here is an example of a basic arm movement during a grand plié.

You start with arms in the second position. The arms go down to preparatory position during the demi plié. When you move through your deepest point, the arms move back up to the first position, and arrive there when you are back in your demi plié. While stretching the legs, the arms can open again to the second position.

Be careful not to 'swipe' your arms along your thighs. Keep your shoulders above your hips, and your belly button in with lightly activated stomach and buttocks muscles.

Practice your épaulement while your plié. Follow the movements of your arms with your eyes and head.

Bending and stretching are very important and the basis of almost all ballet movements. The plié has the function of setting off to the next movement or landing from a movement. It also ensures a smooth and beautiful transition from one to the other.
So, let's practice it well!

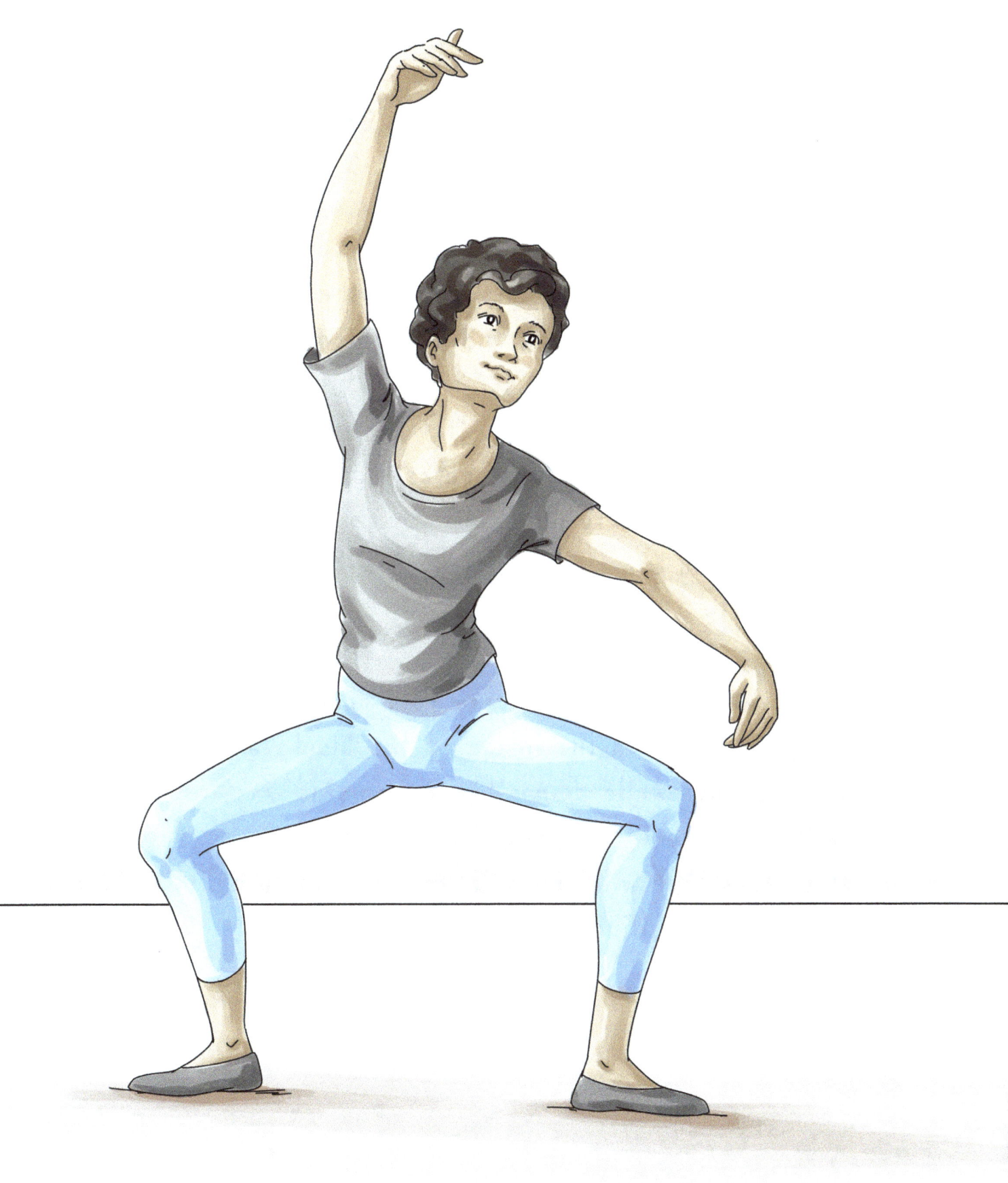

Chapter 8: élevé and relevé

The French verbs relever and élever both mean to raise.
What does that mean for a ballet movement?
I'm going to tell you how I learned it.

Stand in the first foot position and rise on the ball of your foot. This is élevé. You go straight up and straight down.

Stand in the first position again on flat feet. Now you make a demi plié. From this demi plié you push yourself up on the balls of your feet. Like you were going to jump, but you're not going up in the air. This is a relevé. You can come back down with straight legs or go down in a demi plié.

You can do élevé and relevé in every foot position you want. Think of your basic position and the image of the blocks all nicely stacked on top of each other while doing this movement.

A good élevé or relevé will help you to jump and turn well, and have beautiful, smooth transitions while you dance.

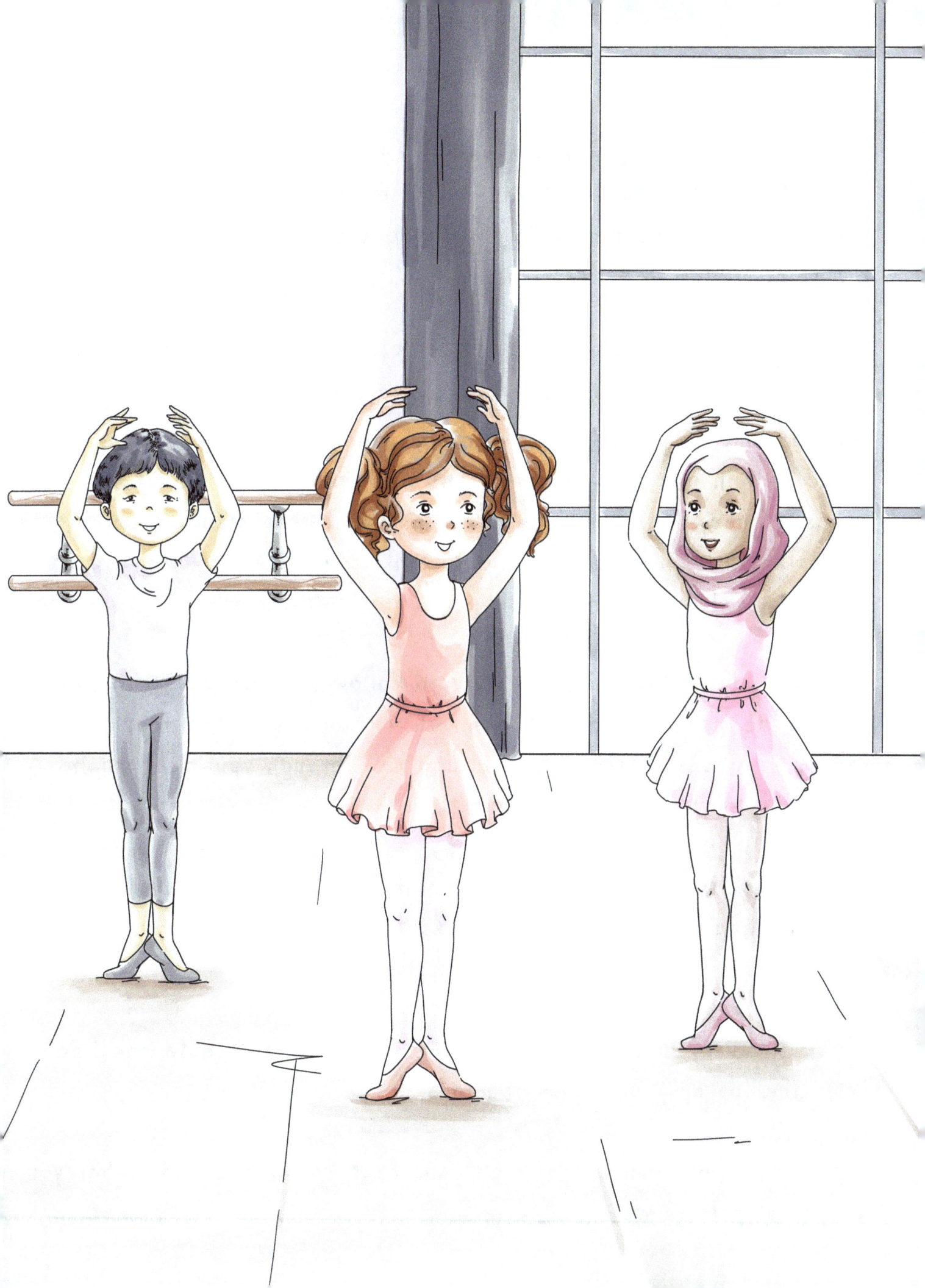

Chapter 9: Tendu

Tendu comes from the French verb tendre. One of the meanings is to stretch. In ballet specifically it is a movement to stretch your legs and feet. That can be to the front, side or back. It is used as the start or link to ballet steps.

Let's try from our first foot position. Start moving your leg to the front in a direct line coming from your heel. Keep the toes on the floor as long as possible and then go ahead and stretch out the whole foot in line with your leg. The movement starts under your hip bones, so keep your hips and pelvis in place. Keep standing upright on your standing leg, be careful not to sink into the hip or you will have difficulties closing the leg back in.

With a tendu to the side, you want to follow one line out from your middle toe. Try to keep your turn out. The inside of the foot is facing the front. Again, go ahead and roll through your foot when you move to full stretch and back in.

To the back is tricky. It is easy to sink in and move your pelvis. We need to start from the foot, keep the turn out and go in one straight line out and back in. Nicely done!

Tip 1: In every direction you want to make sure to create one line from the top of your leg to you toes.

Tip 2: the more you can stretch your feet, the better and higher you will be able to jump.

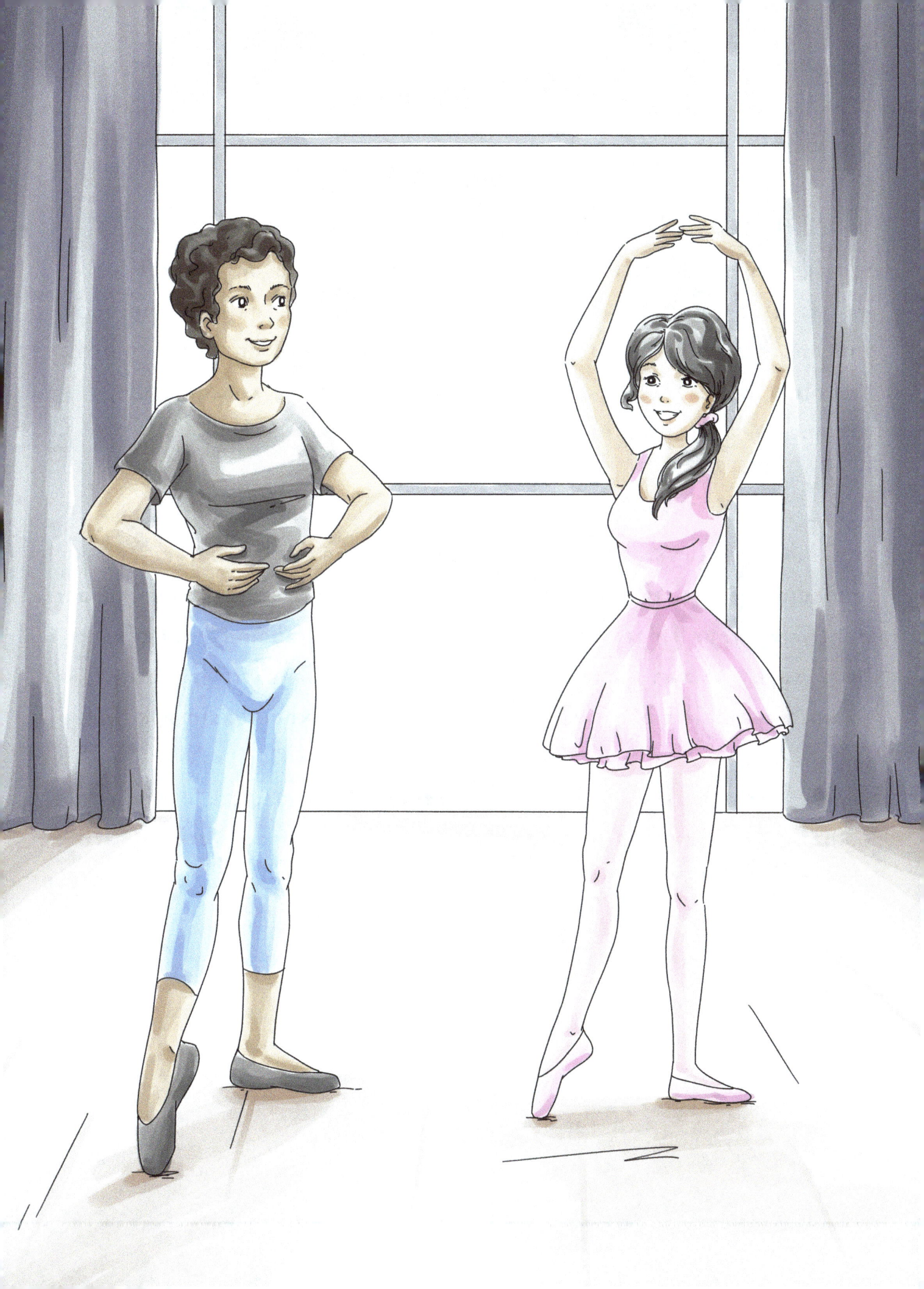

Chapter 10: Why do we dance at the barre?

We start class at the barre. The barre is there to help you out, should you need extra help balancing and dancing on one leg. We practice ballet movements and steps with one half of the body, and one hand on the barre. Then turn around and do it again with the other half. This is done to learn and practice coordination, balance en get stronger and leaner muscles.

Stand next to the barre and put your arms in the second arm position. Now lower one arm so your hand meets the barre. You will immediately feel if you are too close or too far away from the barre. Gently lay your fingers on the barre, without grabbing hold of it. Have soft, relaxed fingers, wrist, and elbow. Check if the arm is not forward or to the back. This has an effect on your basic position.

Try to learn to rely on your own core and leg muscles to stand. Sometimes I see arm and hand muscles flexing and working hard on a barre, and that is not necessary and will not help you improve your balance.

That's it! Looking good!

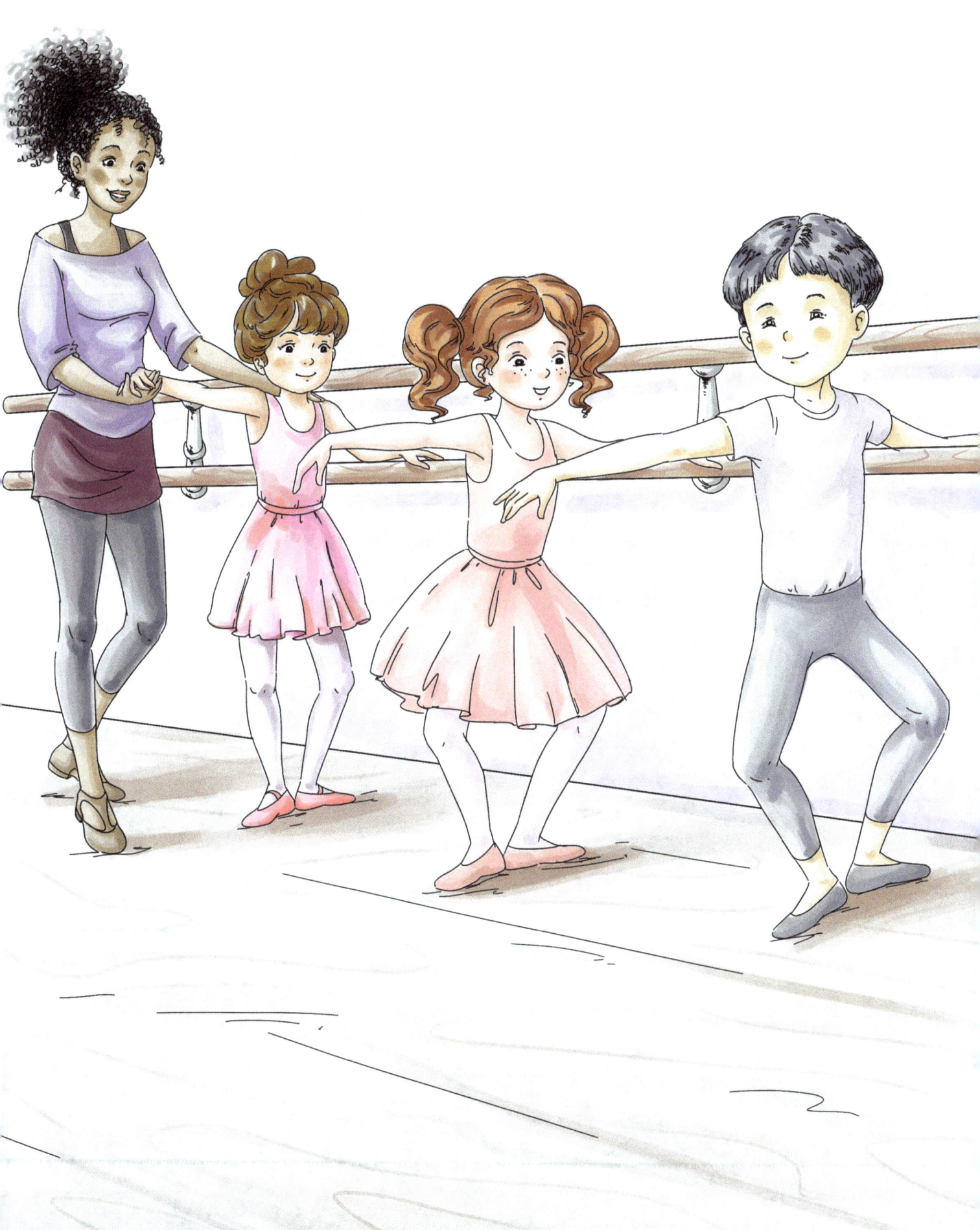

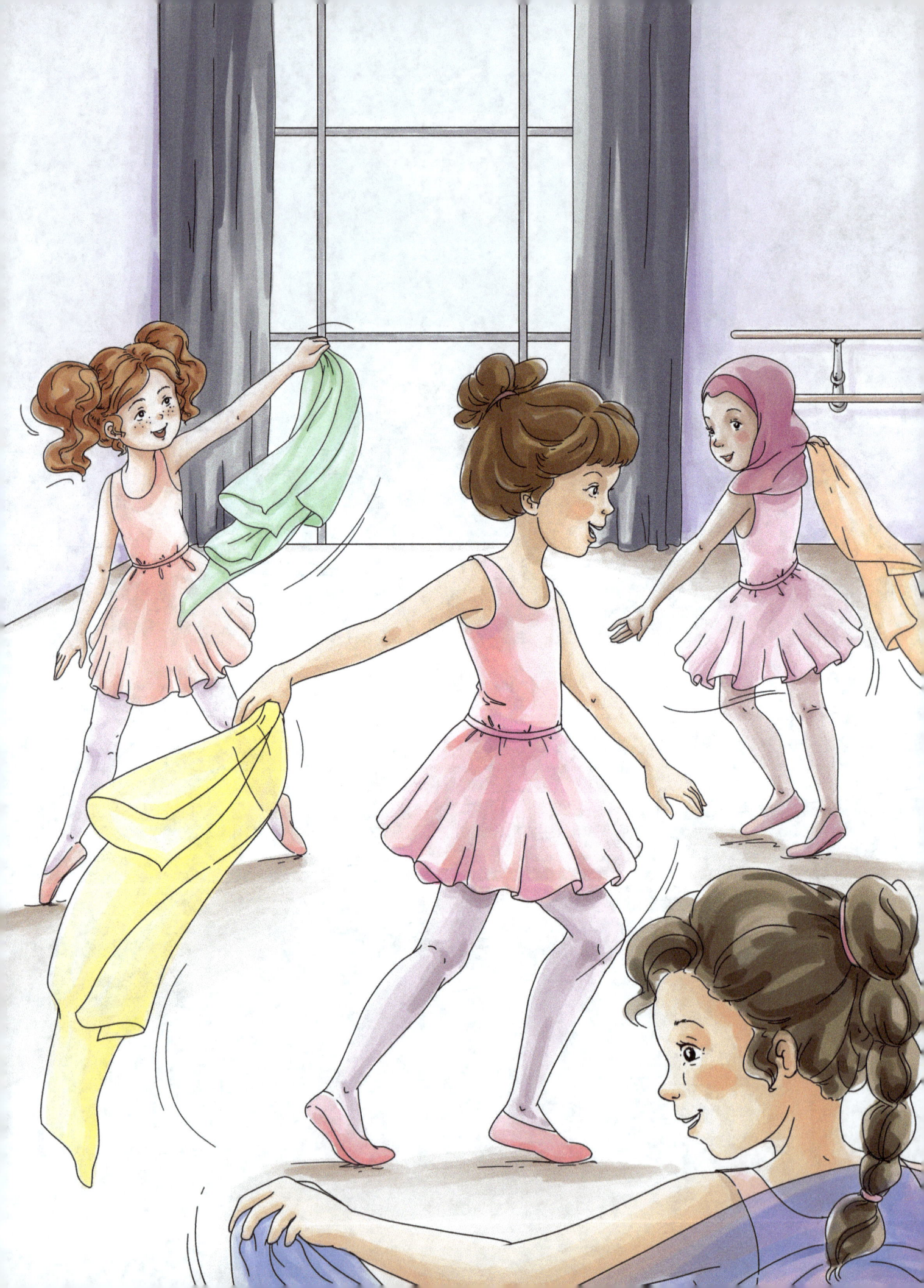

Chapter II: Dancing to and with the music.

In the ballet class you will dance to music. This music will help you dance the ballet steps to the fullest. It will vary in tempo, sometimes slow and sometimes fast. It will also vary in dynamics, being softer or stronger. Go ahead and really listen to the music, it will help you a lot in dancing the steps.

You will learn to get information for your dance in the introduction of the music. The tempo, the dynamics, the beat, and the measure. It will improve your musicality when you know when to start and finish and when to come into the music when you are dancing in turns.

An important part of the ballet class will also be improvisation. Your teacher will tell you a story or give you a theme and choose music for you to dance to. And sometimes you may choose the music yourself. With that story or theme in mind and the music you will start to dance and make up your own steps and ballet sequence. This will help you listen to music, react to an atmosphere, and understand which ballet steps are appropriate to which mood and moment.

Chapter 12:
Dancing in the middle and out of the corner of the room.

During the ballet class you will also dance in the middle of the room, in front of the mirror. All you have practiced at the barre with one body halve, will now be danced with the whole body. This will take better balancing on one leg and coordination of arms and legs.
You will use the mirror to check if your posture and lines are as good as you feel they are. Your teacher will also keep an eye on you to make sure you are dancing correctly and safely.

Standing in front of the mirror with the whole group will teach you to become aware and mindful of your surroundings. In the ballet world we call that 'spacing'. It means you will know and feel where the other dancers are in the space you occupy.

You can dance in a circle, rectangle or in rows. And with dancing from one corner to the other corner across the floor you will learn to dance in patters and together in small groups. There is a lot of variety, and it is very fun to do.

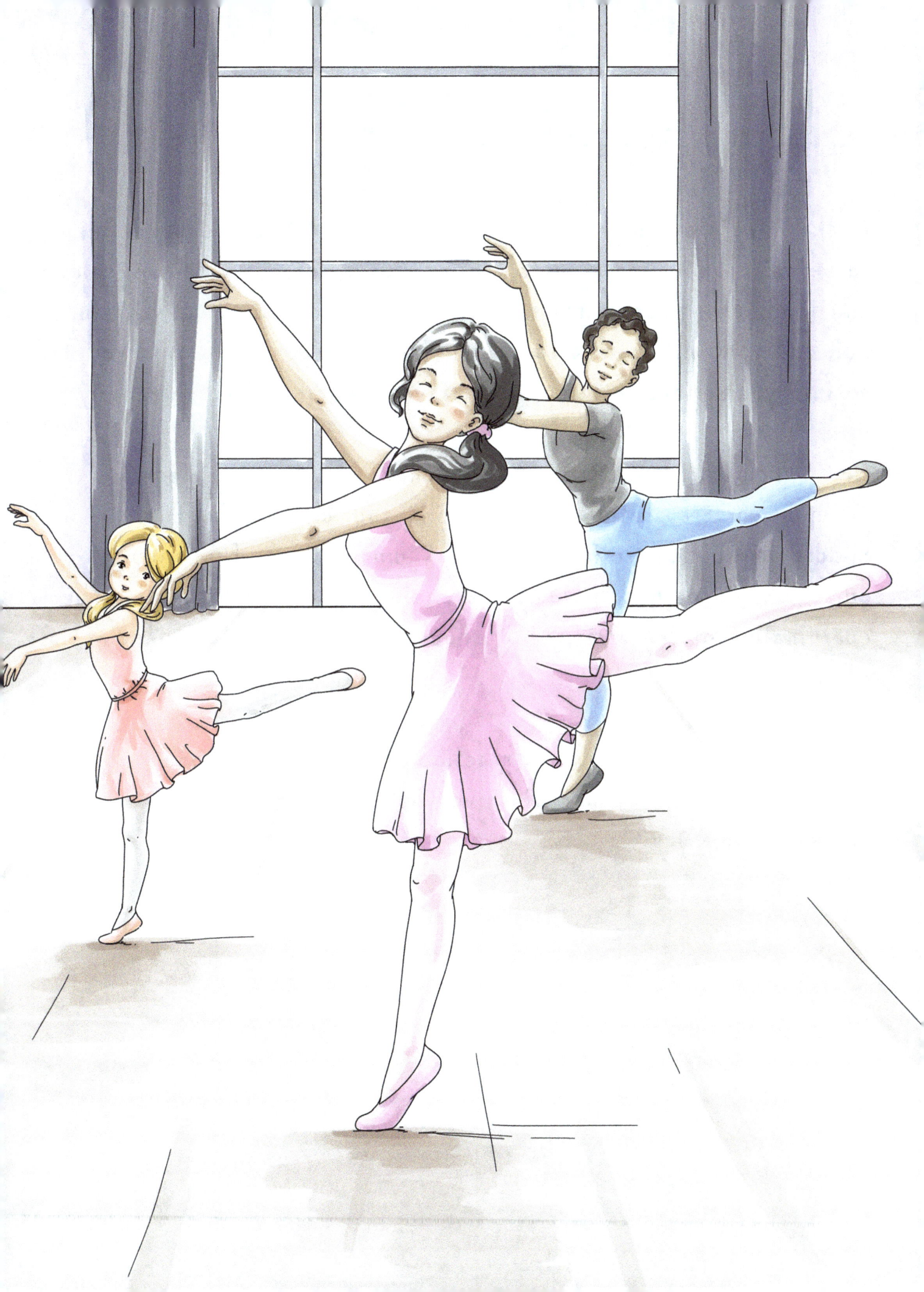

Chapter 13: Jumping and Turning

In the middle of our ballet journey together, I told you about the three basic ballet movements. These movements (plié, élevé, relevé and tendu) we need to master correctly. If you let go of your turn out, and your plié is incorrect, your jump will go poorly. And you can't go into your pirouette (turn). But if you can, it will go splendidly.

See a jump or turn as a whole sequence. They have a clear beginning or preparation, usually a plié and, or a tendu. There is a middle or main attraction, the actual jump or turn. This requires your guts. Just do it. And there is the ending, again usually a plié. The coordination of the arms, neck, shoulders, and head (épaulement) are going to help you.

At the end of class, you will practice this with your group and teacher. Your teacher will give you feedback and tips on how to improve.

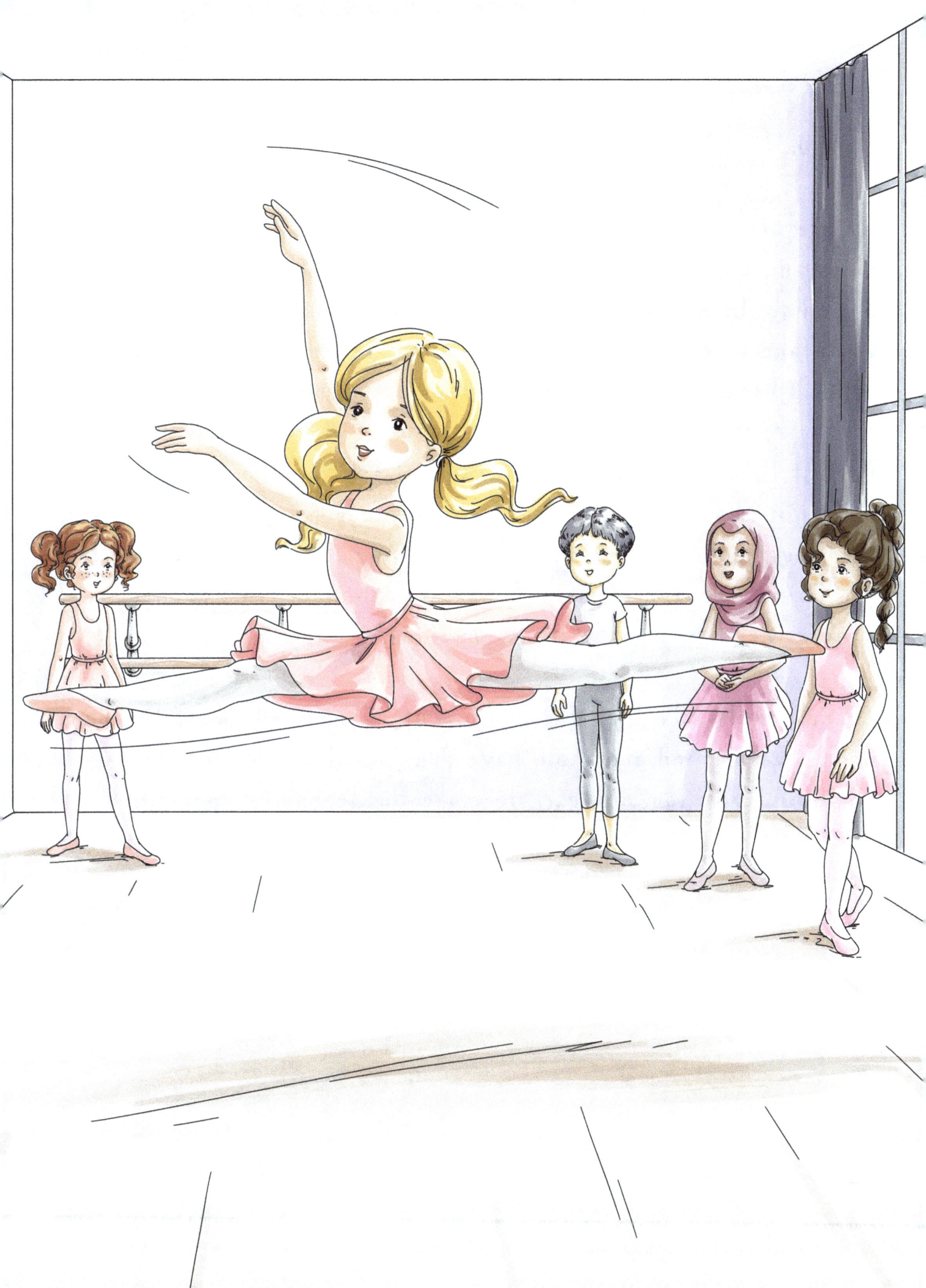

Conclusion:

We are at the end of this story. There are so many beautiful ballet steps and dances. But I promised you we would talk about the very beginning, the basics. Remember? And that is what we have done. Learn and practice and you will see that learning more advanced ballet steps will become easier because you understand the basis.

My last tips: Listen to your teacher and ask questions. Above all try, move your body, and have fun. The only way for your body to learn the movements is to do it. Just do it. And it is perfectly fine that you do not succeed at first. Even very talented, professional ballet dancers need to practice. It is how it is.

All new skills take time to master. But if you really want to, then don't give up. And above all, have fun. Ballet is for everyone, so use all the information you learn to make the technique your own.

Bye!

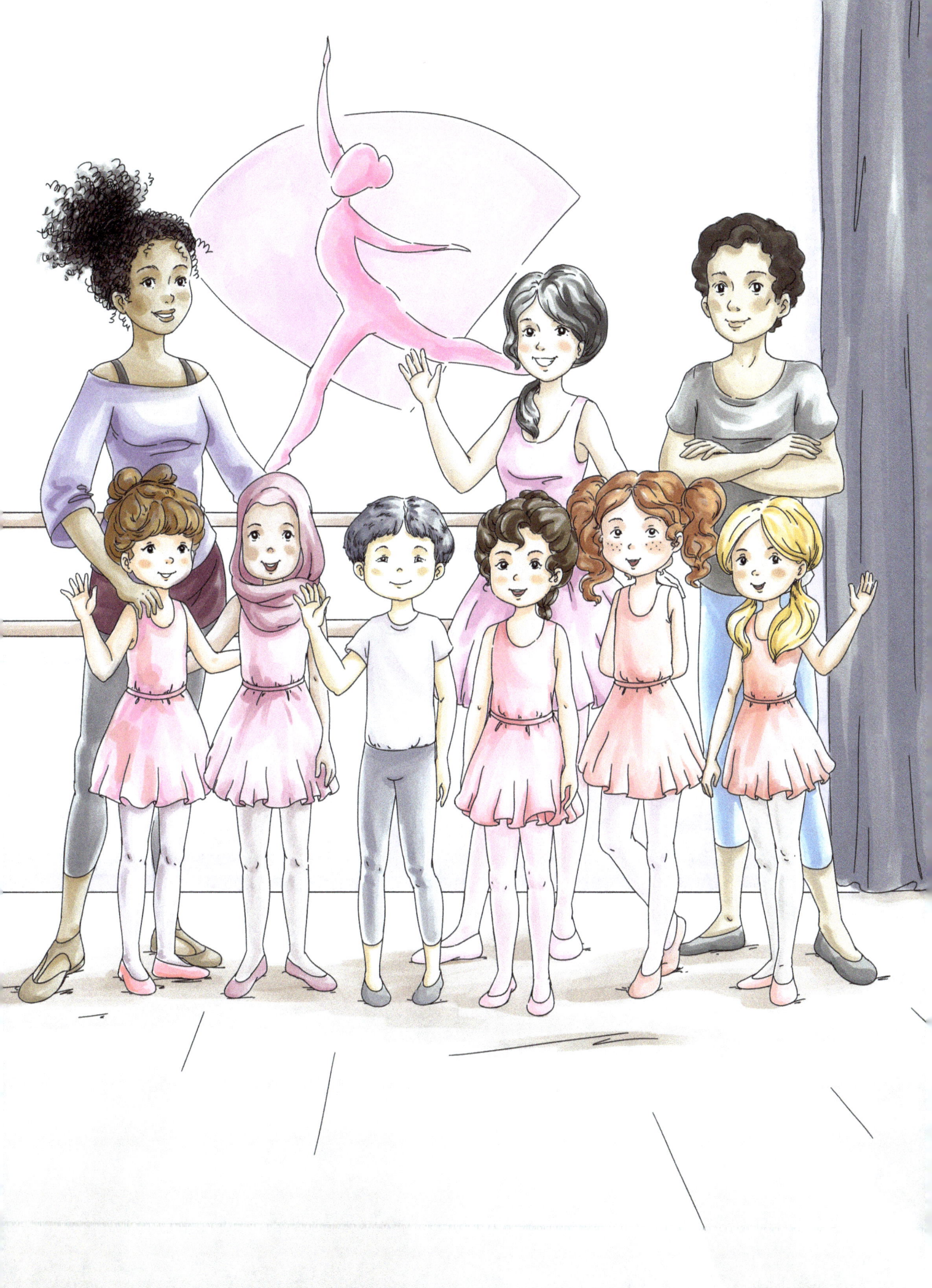

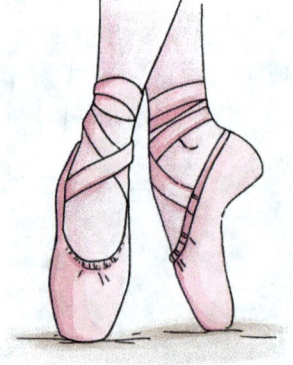

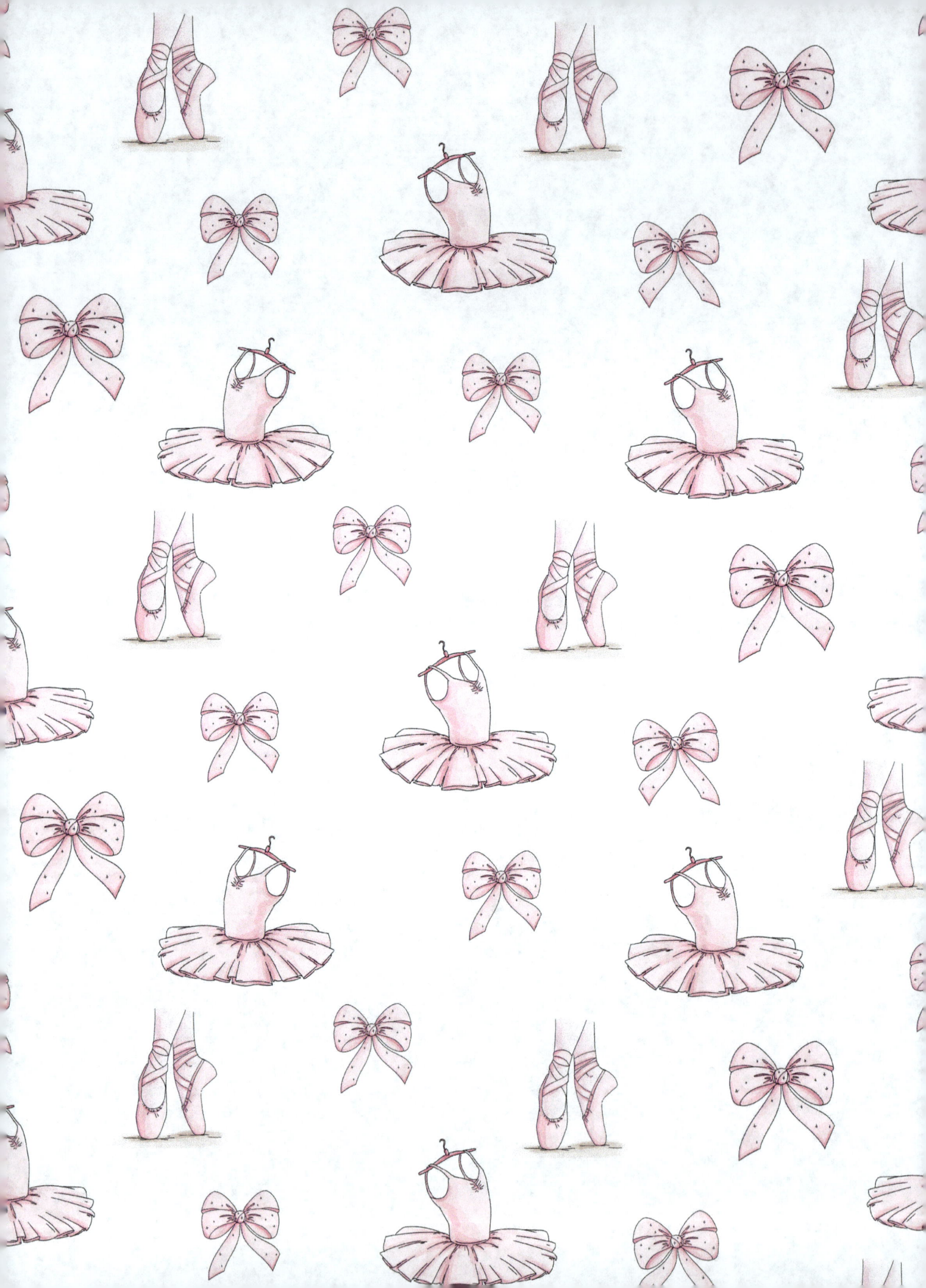

www.ingramcontent.com/pod-product-compliance
Lightning Source LLC
LaVergne TN
LVHW061958070526
838199LV00060B/4190